Group Therapy
For Cancer and Serious Illness

Treatment Manual

Stacey Y. Scott, PsyD
Licensed Clinical Psychologist

Scott, Stacey (2008) ISBN 978-0-6152-0083-5
from Scott, S. (2003). *Faith supportive group therapy and symptom reduction in Christian breast cancer patients.* Ann Arbor, MI, Proquest Information and Learning. UMI Microform 3075442.

Contents

This manual is adapted from Appendix C of *Faith Supportive Group Therapy and Symptom Reduction in Christian Breast Cancer Patients*, presented to the faculty of the Doctoral Psychology Program of Regent University, Virginia Beach, Virginia, in November of 2001 in partial fulfillment of the requirements for the degree: Doctorate of Psychology. It is dedicated to my committee, Dr. John Spencer, Dr. Holiday Rondeau, and Warren Withrow, M.Div, particularly to Dr. John Spencer who first proposed the project to me and who helped to shape my career in caring for cancer and serious illness.

My work with cancer and serious illness began and continues in memory of my mother, Charlotte Rainey Scott, who was diagnosed with late-stage ovarian cancer in August, 1993. She died 6 weeks after her diagnosis, but her inspiration and character continue to influence my work with this very special population.

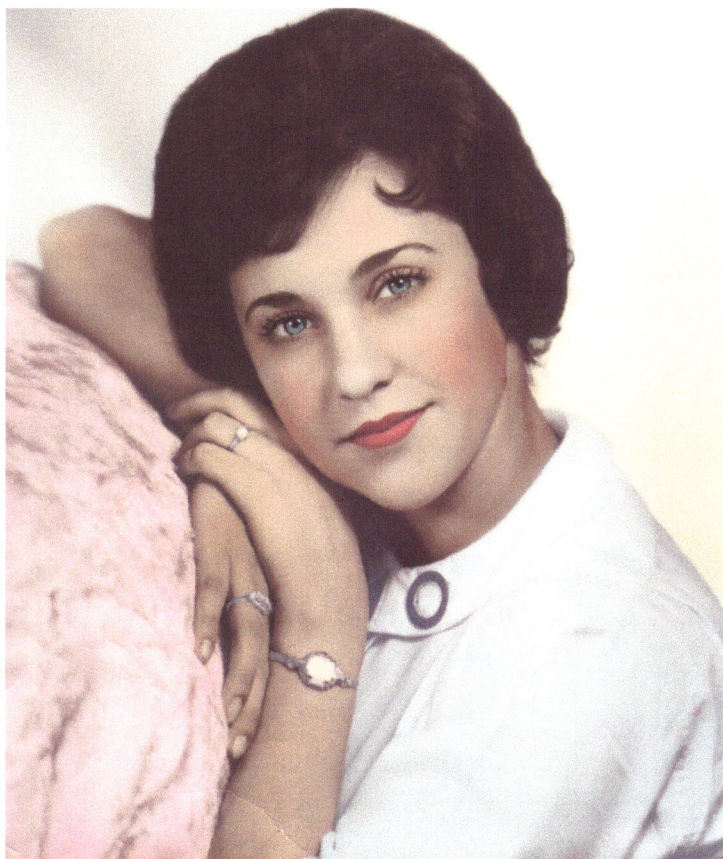

Charlotte Rainey Scott, January 15th, 1943 - September 7th, 1993

Manual Content:
Overview of Session Format

Overview of Session Format

The sessions in this manual are arranged so that the topics, agenda, and materials needed for each session are grouped together. Each session is designed to be approximately 90 minutes in length and is closed with a relaxation exercise lasting from 10 to 20 minutes. Handouts, scripts for relaxation, and any additional therapist information is included immediately following the corresponding session.

Each session includes the following:

Session Number

Subject

Agenda
- Agenda items
- Agenda items

Materials Needed:
1. Material
2. Material

Notes for facilitator describing the section and purpose, including any areas to be aware of in the group process.

Time Allotted: (listed here)

This area will include the therapist's script, instructions for presenting material to participants, or explanations of a procedure, skill, or area of instruction to describe to participants. This can be read verbatim in a relaxed style or can be paraphrased in the style comfortable to the facilitator. If read in the facilitator's own style, be careful to remain within the parameters of the treatment and to be consistent with the session goals, focus, and therapeutic framework.

Session 1

Subject: Introduction of participants and explanation of therapeutic approach

Agenda:

- Greeting and introduction of facilitator(s) and group members
- Explanation of therapeutic approach
- Group Guidelines (handout)
- Handout of Session dates and topics
- Rapport building: sharing reasons for joining group and what participants hope to gain from group
- Breathing exercise

Materials Needed:
1. Handouts of session dates and topics (list any dates that you will not be meeting due to holiday, vacation, etc.)
2. Handouts of general group guidelines
3. Dry Erase board or flip chart
4. Markers, eraser

- Greeting

Facilitator greets participants and provides rationale for cognitive behavioral approach

Time Allotted: 20 Minutes

"Thank you for agreeing to participate in this group experience. The group will meet once a week for an hour and ½ for eight sessions. The purpose of this group is to help you to cope with the emotions, thoughts, and changes in your lives as a result of your diagnosis and treatment. You will have time each week to share what you are feeling or experiencing and to learn and practice exercises that have proven to be effective in dealing with and reducing stress responses, tension, anxiety, depression, and physical discomfort.

By participating in the sessions actively and practicing the techniques at home, it is hoped that you will be able to gain greater coping skills and a sense of control over what is happening in your body and with your emotions. One benefit of group therapy is the social support of others who are facing similar challenges. Social support is one of the leading ways of coping reported by patients facing serious illness."

"I'd like to tell you a little about myself. My name is _____ and I am a (area of practice, credentials, license, experience, etc.). I'm going to spend a little time explaining the approaches that were chosen for this group therapy program. The approach combines Cognitive Behavioral Therapy with stress management and coping skills. Cognitive Behavior Therapy is a well-known and very effective intervention for depression and anxiety and operates from the premise that our thoughts, feelings, and behaviors are interrelated, and that if we can learn to identify our thoughts, we can find ways to reduce distress by targeting certain types of thoughts for change. Even subtle changes in what we automatically tell ourselves can have an effect on our emotions. Cognitive Behavioral Therapy is supported by years of research on people struggling with difficult emotions. The approach will also focus on behaviors that cue certain types of emotions and those that follow certain emotions. All emotions have action urges and thoughts. If we can change the thought or action, we can often experience a change in emotion.

According to this model, negative emotions (those you don't want, that aren't helping you, or are getting in the way of you being effective) have specific types of thoughts that accompany or trigger them. Sadness generally involves thoughts of loss. The loss may be very real, anticipated, feared, or imagined. What we are saying to ourselves about the loss is key. Although there are certain types of thinking that can elicit a negative mood, it is important to differentiate between thoughts and feelings that are warranted, understandable, and justified by the situation. This approach does not advocate or teach us to gloss over, diminish, or change valid responses to actual situations, or that difficult emotions can be avoided. Grief is a human reaction to loss; fear is a human reaction to a threat to life, health, or wellbeing. There is no expectation for people to be happy, positive, or free of emotional distress as an end result. There is evidence that emotional distress or pain can be reduced by use of these strategies.

These strategies can help you to learn to recognize and cope with your feelings in unquestionably difficult situations so that we reduce the negative effects of prolonged stress and emotional strain on your body and mind. The relaxation and coping strategies will help you to activate systems in your body that counter the stress response, including the parasympathetic nervous system and positive endorphins that accompany pleasant events and help to lift mood and improve our quality of life.

Does anyone have any questions?"

- Group Guidelines

Facilitator will discuss the format and the general principles for group interactions.

Time Allotted: 10 minutes

Everyone will have an opportunity to share, however the sessions will be conducted according to a pre-determined set of topics and exercises. It is important to address feelings and experiences but the purpose of this group will not be best served by spending the entire period in open discussion. There will be weekly topics and discussion around those topics as well as practice of the techniques that will be introduced so that you will be able to use them outside of the sessions. There will always be time each week to share thoughts and feelings about your diagnosis and what is going on in your lives. We do need to set some guidelines for group discussion.

General principles are:

1. Always let whoever is talking finish speaking before responding.
2. Let the therapist worry about guiding time in discussion - everyone will get an opportunity to speak but sometimes a personal situation that is relevant to the group's purpose might be explored in more detail.
3. Try to attend each session and let me know if you cannot make it. Group members will grow to depend on each other's support and presence in the meetings so it is important not only for the process but also for the other members that you attend.
4. We will need to start and finish on time. If you feel seriously distressed at the end of group and are uncomfortable leaving things where they are until next time, please talk to me about it after the session.
5. Being supportive of each other can be accomplished by just listening even though you might feel pulled to give other members solutions. Be aware that statements beginning with: "I think you should…." (or a similar remark) imply a judgment and will not be as helpful. It <u>will</u> be helpful to share personal experience that relates to what other group members are going through.
6. Confidentiality is essential. Please do not repeat personal information about other group members to those outside of group. It is fine to discuss your own progress and group topics with others; however be careful not to give any information that could identify other members.

▪   Introduction of participants, reasons for joining group and expectations.

Facilitator will open the floor for group introductions and sharing.
Time allotted: 30 minutes

I would like for everyone to introduce him or herself and say whatever you are comfortable sharing concerning your diagnosis and what you hope to gain from the group experience.
(Model appropriate interaction by reflective listening and supportive statements.)

▪   Breathing Exercise

Facilitator will introduce breathing relaxation technique and lead group in breathing exercise.
Time allotted: 15 minutes

I'd like to close with a short breathing exercise that we will use during some of our relaxation techniques. Please sit comfortably with both feet on the floor and your spine as straight as possible and breath as you normally do.
(Wait for members to arrange posture)

Now place one hand on the spot that seems to rise and fall as you inhale and exhale. If the spot is in your chest, move it down to your abdomen. Breathe in slowly and then exhale so that your abdomen is the area rising and falling. This makes the best use of the lower part of your lungs. People who are nervous tend to breathe quicker, shallow breaths using their upper chest. If it is possible, breathe in through your nose and out through your mouth. Spend a minute or two breathing slowly and feeling your abdomen rise and fall. Now, as you breathe out through your mouth relax your jaw and let it fall open a little and breathe out as though you were blowing air on a frosty window. Continue to breathe in and out slowly, relaxing your jaw and mouth as you exhale.
 (Model and continue for approximately 10 breaths)

You can practice this breathing exercise anytime. I encourage each of you to try this exercise when you are feeling tense during the week and see how it works for you.

•   Closing   ***Time allotted: 10 minutes***

Facilitator completes closing with Session Dates and Topics handout and emergency contact number.

Session Dates and Topics

1. Introductory session and overview	Date:_____
2. Initial and Current Reactions to Your Diagnosis	Date: _____
3. Medical Questions and Introduction to Thought Charting	Date: _____
4. Thought Charting, Thinking Styles, and Reframing	Date: _____
5. The Reaction of Family Members and Others to Your Diagnosis	Date: _____
6. Self-Image and Intimate Relationships	Date: _____
7. Establishing New Goals	Date: _____
8. Summing Up and Reviewing Coping Skills	Date: _____

<u>Group Guidelines</u>

- Confidentiality is important. What goes on in the group stays in the group. Please do not identify group members or their discussions outside of group time. You can talk about your own experiences in the group to others, but be mindful not to discuss someone else's experience.
- Discussions will be paced by the group leader. This is a therapeutic group with certain points that will be covered in order to process feelings and build coping skills. Since the format is different than a "support group" conversational or social subjects will be gently guided back on task by the group leader.
- Attending each session is important. The coping skills build upon each other, and others will grow to depend on each person's unique contribution to the group. Please notify the group leader if you will have to miss a session.
- Your participation is voluntary. If at any time you decide that you no longer want to participate, you may stop attending. In this case, please consider attending for a final session so that group members can say goodbye.

Emergency contact number:

Session 2

Subject: Your First Emotional Reaction to the Diagnosis

Agenda:

- The first emotional reaction to the diagnosis.
- Cognitive Messages.
- Discussion throughout how patients are feeling and thinking about God.
- Legitimize and validate the emotions of the participants.
- Progressive muscle relaxation technique.
- Closing

Materials Needed
1. Flip chart or dry-erase board 2. Markers 3. Handouts of feeling words (One per participant). 4. 3-column worksheet for identifying negative self-talk associated with emotional distress (One per participant). 5. Breathing and relaxation script.

- The First Emotional Reaction to the Diagnosis

Facilitator will introduce and lead a discussion on the participants' first feelings about their diagnosis.

Time Allotted: 15 minutes

> In this session we are going to focus on your feelings, specifically the feelings you had at the time of your diagnosis and the feelings you have now about your cancer (or serious illness "_____") and treatment. I'm going to ask each of you to share your feelings. While you are talking about them I'm going to write them on a chart (or dry-erase board) so that we can see and identify your emotions. Anything goes, so feel free to express yourselves openly. If you have feelings that seem different from the others being expressed that's O.K; there is no right or wrong way to feel in these circumstances.
>
> (***Ask for a volunteer to begin or pick a person by saying...***) Let's start here with _____ and work around. When you first received your diagnosis, what were you feeling?

> (**Write feeling words down on the chart in a column as they are expressed. Verbally acknowledge similar and different feelings among participants.**)
> Now that we have a picture of the feelings, let's look at who or what they are directed towards. (**Repeat the feeling words and ask each member respectively...**)
> For example, if you are feeling angry, the anger is about, at, towards...?
> (**Write their answers on the chart next to their feelings.**)

Example:

Emotions	About or towards
anger	cancer
ignored	doctor; nursing staff

(Discuss)

- Cognitive Messages

Facilitator will lead a discussion on the automatic thoughts that are connected to the feelings in reaction to their diagnosis.

Time Allotted: 30 minutes

> The next step is to try and identify what you are automatically thinking when you feel these emotions, for example a common thought under feelings of anger might be, "This is unfair", or "Why me?"
>
> What are some of the things you are <u>thinking</u> when you feel angry, sad, and upset?
>
> (**List the thoughts that are generated next to who or what the feelings were directed.**)
> (**Try to guide members to place thoughts into "I" messages. For example: "There is nothing I can do about the situation"; "I don't deserve this"; I am being punished"; etc.**)

Example:

Emotions	About or Towards	Thoughts or Beliefs
Anger	cancer (or illness)	I don't want this to be happening

- Legitimize or Validate the Emotions

Facilitator will refer back to the emotions listed and validate the feelings to let participants know and understand that the emotions they are experiencing are not abnormal in light of their diagnosis and experiences.

Time Allotted: 15 minutes

It is important for you to know that you are experiencing <u>normal reactions</u> to a situation that is not within our normal set of life circumstances. The emotions that you are feeling and the thoughts of unfairness and helplessness are just as real and distressing as the presence of the cancer. Just as the doctors work to reduce or eliminate cancer, you can work to reduce feelings of distress that are causing additional symptoms such as anxiety, sadness, irritability, and tension. <u>Actively participating</u> in your treatment can help.

In the next few sessions we will go over strategies for building coping and participation such as correct diet, physical activity, reframing negative thinking, learned relaxation, and guided imagery. We will also address coping benefits of your faith life and will utilize spiritual strategies whenever appropriate. These techniques are designed to help you deal with the feelings associated with your diagnosis, not to discount or eliminate those feelings. It is normal to feel extreme emotions in the face of an extreme situation. What you **do** to cope with the situation is the key.

I'm going to pass around a worksheet for you to do over the next week. It will give you a chance to identify other feelings and automatic thoughts or beliefs just like we did today. Please use the worksheet when distressing emotions arise and bring it next time. (Hand out one worksheet per participant). Do you have any questions about this worksheet? **(Answer any questions on the use of the worksheet columns.)**

- Progressive Muscle Relaxation Techniques

Time Allotted: 20 minutes

We're going to do another relaxation technique starting with deep breathing and then moving into muscle relaxation. You may find this exercise helpful in reducing physical and emotional tension. Let's learn this type of relaxation by trying it out. I will be directing you to tense and release specific muscle groups, but **if you are feeling pain or discomfort in any part of your body, please feel free to follow along with breathing only. Do not do any part of this exercise if it causes pain.** Please follow my directions as I read aloud.

(Facilitator follows relaxation script for session 3.)

You can practice this outside of the group by starting with deep breathing and then tensing and relaxing your muscles. Try to practice this week when you feel tense and remember to record your thoughts and feelings on the worksheet.

- Closing

Facilitator will close the session by asking if there are any questions about the progressive muscle relaxation exercise, and assigning exercises to practice at home.

Time Allotted: 15 minutes

Thank you for your participation this session. I look forward to seeing each of you next week. Please try to complete at least a little bit of your feelings and thoughts worksheet. You may find this very helpful in becoming familiar with the connection between your feelings and thinking. Also, try out your new muscle relaxation exercise at least one time before you return for next session.

Breathing and Relaxation Exercise

The basic premise of the muscle relaxation we are going to do now is that it is physically impossible for your body to be tense when you are in a state of relaxation. This technique identifies the difference between a tense and relaxed state and gives you an option for reducing physiological distress. We will be working on activating the Parasympathetic Nervous System, the opposite of the Fight or Flight response. Many people find that, when they reduce physical arousal, their thoughts and emotions also follow and become less intense.

Facilitator should read this script aloud, slowly allowing a pause between instructions, particularly when it reads "Practice this for a moment" or "hold the tension". Modeling the technique throughout the session is also very helpful since some clients will not feel comfortable keeping their eyes closed.

1. Sit comfortably with your feet on the floor and arms to your sides.

2. Pay attention to your breathing. Breathe in more slowly, take air in through your nose and exhale through your mouth. As you breathe in, your chest should not rise. Correct breathing will go to the diaphragm-your stomach should be the base for the air. Practice this for a moment. Now, as you exhale through your mouth pretend that you are blowing on a spoonful of hot soup or that you are blowing on a frosty window. It should not be forced. You can also pretend that you are deflating.

    Practice this for a moment.
    Keep breathing comfortably and slowly.
    If you feel comfortable, close your eyes as you continue to breathe. Let yourself become quiet and still. It may help to think the word "calm" to yourself as you breathe out, or to imagine a color of fresh air as you breathe in, and a color for the stress that you exhale.

3. Now tense your toes and feet and hold the tension. Feel the muscles working to hold the tension. Now relax your feet. Notice that they feel lighter. Continue to breathe in through the nose and out through the mouth.

4. Now tense your lower legs, knees and thighs and hold the tension. Notice the strain and the effort you are using. Now let go of the tension, relaxing your lower legs, knees, and thighs. Notice as you are breathing that your legs and feet are light and relaxed.

5. Now tense your lower abdomen. Hold the tension...and release. The lower half of your body is peaceful, heavy as if sleeping.

6. Now tense your chest and upper arm muscles. Notice the tension. Relax your chest and upper arms, continuing to breathe deep, calming breaths centered on the diaphragm.

7. Now tense the upper back and shoulders, raising your shoulders towards your ears. Hold the tension. Now let your shoulders drop and let go of the muscles in your shoulders and upper back. You notice that your shoulders, back, abdomen, thighs, legs, and feet are heavy and relaxed.

8. Now tense the muscles of your neck and lower face, tightening your jaw, mouth, and chin. Hold it for a moment, and release the tension. Notice the difference. Let your jaw go loose so that your upper and lower teeth are not clenched. Continue to relax.

9. Now tense your forehead and eye muscles and hold the tension. Continue to breathe slowly. Now let go of the tension relaxing your forehead, eyebrows, eyes, and head. Study the feeling of relaxation in your body. As you continue to breathe slowly, you feel completely at peace and rest. Your body is heavy, almost as if it is sinking into the chair. You think about lifting your arm but it is too heavy. You are relaxed and calm.

10. As you continue to breathe, slowly begin to notice the sounds around you in the room as you remain relaxed. As I count backward in a moment you will open your eyes and return to the room feeling a continued sense of calm throughout your whole body.

   4   3   2   1   Open your eyes and stretch.

Checklist of Distressing Feelings

Feeling low	Sad
Self-critical	Useless
Worthless	Afraid
Incapable	Numb
Hopeless	Preoccupied
Obsession	Fear
Hating my life	Disorganized
Helpless	Suspicious
Anxious	Empty; void
Apathetic	Like a failure
Unbearable	Apprehensive
Tense	Dead inside
Agitated	Quiet
Miserable	Shock
Withdrawn	Alone
Guilty	Grief

Thought Charting

Situation	Emotions/Feelings	Thoughts/Beliefs

Notes:

Session 3

Subject: Education: Medical Questions, Diet, and Treatment Complications

Agenda:

- Sharing questions and information.
- Checking on thoughts and feelings worksheet.
- Relaxation exercise
- Closing.

Materials Needed

1. Literature on diet, side effects of treatment, and paper for   recording questions.
2. Flip chart or dry-erase board.
3. Markers.
4. 3-column worksheets. (One per participant)
5. Handout of common types of cognitive distortions.

- Education: Medical Information

Introduce the topic of taking an active role in treatment through use of correct diet and physical activity. Questions can be asked about fears, concerns over treatment effects and cancer. This should not take up more than 20-30 minutes.

Time Allotted: 30 minutes

Hello everyone. Today I would like for you to think about any health questions you may have in regard to your diagnosis or about how to take an active role in your treatment through the use of correct diet and physical activity. Please take a few moments to think of or write down some questions that you may want to ask. We can also discuss question about any fears, concerns about treatment and about cancer itself. (Wait about 2-3 minutes for participants to formulate questions.) Who would like to start?

(Facilitate a discussion including questions and answers on any of the above stated topics. Be prepared to process any feelings of anger or frustration with health care and medical services during the discussion. You may do this by allowing to let the participant voice their feelings and validating them, while encouraging empathy and understanding of the demands and limitations of health care providers.)

Before moving on to thought-charting, make sure to have written down questions that the group might want answered. These can be compiled and given to an oncology nurse or professional for clarification and answers. Share the results with the group in a later session.

- Checking on Thoughts/Feelings Worksheet

Facilitator will lead a discussion on the thoughts and feelings identified throughout the last week in regard to completing the 3-column worksheet.
Have the flip-chart or dry-erase board ready for reviewing and sharing the feelings and automatic thoughts the group is willing to share. Help the group to rephrase the automatic thoughts and beliefs into "I" messages.

Time Allotted: 30 minutes

We're going to return to the feelings and thoughts that we talked about last time. Would anyone like to share an example of what you recorded last week?

(Facilitator writes examples on the chart in column form, leaving room for a third column:)
Feelings   Thoughts/beliefs about self
_____)

Which thoughts seem to be less helpful for you and seem to produce the greatest emotional upset?
(Discuss)

Now I am going to pass out a list of common types of thinking styles so that you can start to identify patterns of thinking that you see in yourselves.
(Facilitator goes over the thinking styles and finds examples from the flip chart that correspond to some of the types listed.)

What are some thoughts that might work against your quality of life? How so?
(*Facilitator leads a brief group discussion on the participant's answers.)*

Over the next week, I'd like you to continue to chart your emotions and the thoughts that you have connected to them, but now I'd like you to add which type of thinking style corresponds to the beliefs and thoughts. Try to pick out your own pattern of thinking or identify which types you seem to use most often. Next week we will talk about how negative thoughts affect how you feel and respond to situations, and we will teach you the technique for changing some of the patterns of thinking that aren't helping. This is called cognitive reframing.

> (***Pass out new charts for recording thoughts and feelings adding types of cognitive distortions.***)
>
> Are there any questions regarding the worksheet or the completion of this worksheet? (***Answer any questions on the use of the worksheets.***)

- Closing

Time Allotted: 15 minutes

Facilitator completes closing with a reminder to complete the feeling and thinking worksheet and practice the relaxation techniques.

> This session may not have left as much time for sharing and discussion because we needed to include the health and activity talk, but we will have time in the next few sessions to process your thoughts and feelings. Please continue to practice both deep breathing and muscle relaxation when you feel tense and bring your worksheets in next week so that we can add the next step. I look forward to seeing each of you next session.

Thought Charting

Situation	Feelings	Thoughts

Notes:

Thinking Styles

1. All or nothing thinking: everything is in either/or and black/white categories. If things are not great, they are awful. There is no in-between.

2. Overgeneralization: you see a negative event as carrying over into other situations. This happened before, it will happen again.

3. Mental Filter: of all the information you receive, you choose the negative details and focus on those until your vision of reality is darkened.

4. Disqualifying the Positive: positive experiences are downplayed or rejected for some reason so that you maintain a negative belief even if it is contradicted by everyday experiences.

5. Jumping to Conclusions: you interpret things negatively without enough facts to support your conclusion. This can be done in two ways:
   - Mind Reading: you conclude that someone's intentions or actions towards you are negative
   - Fortune Telling: you predict that things will turn out badly and feel convinced that your prediction will occur.

6. Magnification, Catastrophizing, or Minimization: you exaggerate negative events by giving them greater importance or viewing them as a catastrophy, or you shrink positive events and characteristics so that they don't conflict with your negative focus.

7. Emotional Reasoning: you feel something and then label a situation according to your emotions: I feel hurt, so she must have intended to hurt me"

8. Shoulds, Musts, and Oughts: trying to motivate yourself or others with punitive word messages. The emotional consequence is guilt and the feelings elicited will be anger, frustration, and resentment.

9. Labeling and Mislabeling: extreme overgeneralization in which you attach a negative label to yourself or others based on your interpretation of an event: "I'm a loser." or "He's a jerk."

10. Personalization and Blame: you see yourself as the cause of a problem or take on someone else's opinion of you or your situation and give it elevated status.

Session 4

Subject: Review Cognitive Exercise and Relaxation Techniques

Agenda:

- Cognitive charting review; also looking at cognitions relating to faith life.
- Reframing – adding a fourth column.
- Progressive muscle relaxation.
- Closing.

Materials Needed

1. Flip chart or dry-erase board
2. Markers
3. Handouts of 4-column worksheets (One per participant).
4. Breathing and relaxation exercise script

- Cognitive Charting Review

Facilitator will lead a discussion on how the participant's thoughts, beliefs and thinking styles can affect how they feel.

Time Allotted: 30 minutes

We're going to start today by having you get out your thought and feeling charts and talking about the types of thinking styles you were able to identify in yourselves. Who wants to give an example from their worksheet from last week?
(***Write examples on the chart - leave room for reframing column. Begin a time of group discussion by asking the following questions and keeping a time of answering and sharing going among participants.***)

1. Are the thoughts, beliefs, and thinking styles affecting how you feel?

These exercises have been included to help you make a connection between how you interpret situations and how you feel as a result of the interpretation. In order to increase your coping skills and mobilize your resources it is important that you understand the connection so that you can work to change self-messages that may be working against you.

First, we need to identify feelings that are valid responses to negative circumstances, such as fear in response to your diagnosis. These feelings are normal and won't necessarily be targeted for change. We will be looking at additional thoughts that we associate with situations and how those thoughts can aggravate our situations and cause us to feel worse.

Let's look at the examples and see if we can first separate the realistic reactions to situations from the other thoughts and beliefs that we add on.

(Example is: feeling fear after the diagnosis with a thought of the unknown or helplessness is realistic: "what is going to happen to me?" "I don't know how to handle this.", but adding: "I am never going to recover" is a fortune-telling error.)

3. Now that some of the thoughts and beliefs that are additional and unhelpful have been identified, what do we do with them?

- Reframing

Facilitator will introduce the concept of reframing and talk about its practical uses in response to negative styles of thinking.

Time Allotted: 20 minutes

A technique called Reframing is the final step in this process and is something that you can individualize to your personal thinking style. Re-framing involves taking the negative thought or belief and looking at it another way.

Before you reframe it is good to ask the following questions:
1. Is there a larger or different context in which this situation has positive or learning value?
2. What else could be going on besides what I've interpreted?
3. How else could this situation be described?

Reframing doesn't have to be positive, it can simply be less dramatic or it can involve making a neutral statement instead of a negative one. Changing the thought or belief to a less emotionally charged statement will act to bring your level of emotional distress down so that you can more effectively cope with the situation. Again, this is not meant to downplay or eliminate actual distressing events. If someone has just lost a loved one it would be expected that the person would be experiencing extreme grief so re-framing would be inappropriate.

Does everyone see the difference?

What this is intended to do is teach you to identify anticipated or imagined events so that you are not experiencing undue distress over something that hasn't actually happened.

Let's practice reframing with some examples from our list:

(Practice with several examples making sure to watch the time so that you have a good 30 minutes left for the relaxation and closing)
For next week, work on reframing some of the thoughts and beliefs that are connected to distressing feelings. I'm going to give you a new charting handout with the fourth column added. This is the one you will use from now on. If you have trouble coming up with alternative ways to think about a situation or if you get stuck that's O.K., just do the best you can and bring it all in next time.

- Progressive Muscle Relaxation

Facilitator will introduce and lead an exercise in progressive muscle relaxation.
Time Allotted: 20 minutes

We are going to do a more involved form of relaxation that will involve progressively relaxing all of your muscle groups. Progressive Muscle relaxation is a technique used to induce nerve-muscle relaxation. You may find this exercise very helpful in reducing physical and emotional tension. Let's learn this technique by trying it out. Please follow my directions as I read from the script. Get as comfortable as you can, uncross your legs, place your arms at your sides, and start taking deep breaths in through your nose, pausing, and exhaling through your mouth.
(Facilitator follows relaxation script for session 4.)
Please try this exercise during the next week and see how it feels for you outside of the session in a stressful situation.

- Closing

Facilitator completes closing with a reminder to complete the feeling and thinking worksheet and practice the relaxation techniques.

Thank you for your participation in today's session. Please continue to practice relaxing breathing and be sure to try out the new progressive muscle relaxation when you feel tense. Also, please complete a few examples on your new cognitive worksheet, including alternative ways of thinking in the fourth column. Practice reframing, using these alternatives and experience how this technique may change your feelings in distressful situations. Look forward to seeing each of you next session.

Breathing and Relaxation Exercise

The basic premise of the muscle relaxation we are going to do now is that it is physically impossible for your body to be tense when you are in a state of relaxation. This technique identifies the difference between a tense and relaxed state and gives you an option for reducing physiological distress. We will be working on activating the Parasympathetic Nervous System, the opposite of the Fight or Flight response. Many people find that, when they reduce physical arousal, their thoughts and emotions also follow and become less intense.

Facilitator should read this script aloud, slowly allowing a pause between instructions, particularly when it reads "Practice this for a moment" or "hold the tension". Modeling the technique throughout the session is also very helpful since some clients will not feel comfortable keeping their eyes closed.

9. Sit comfortably with your feet on the floor and arms to your sides.

10. Pay attention to your breathing. Breathe in more slowly, take air in through your nose and exhale through your mouth. As you breathe in, your chest should not rise. Correct breathing will go to the diaphragm- your stomach should be the base for the air. Practice this for a moment. Now, as you exhale through your mouth pretend that you are blowing on a spoonful of hot soup or that you are blowing on a frosty window. It should not be forced. You can also pretend that you are deflating.

    Practice this for a moment.
    Keep breathing comfortably and slowly.
    If you feel comfortable, close your eyes as you continue to breathe. Let yourself become quiet and still. It may help to think the word "calm" to yourself as you breathe out, or to imagine a color of fresh air as you breathe in, and a color for the stress that you exhale.

11. Now tense your toes and feet and hold the tension. Feel the muscles working to hold the tension. Now relax your feet. Notice that they feel lighter. Continue to breathe in through the nose and out through the mouth.

12. Now tense your lower legs, knees and thighs and hold the tension. Notice the strain and the effort you are using. Now let go of the tension, relaxing your lower legs, knees, and thighs. Notice as you are breathing that your legs and feet are light and relaxed.

13. Now tense your lower abdomen. Hold the tension...and release. The lower half of your body is peaceful, heavy as if sleeping.

14. Now tense your chest and upper arm muscles. Notice the tension. Relax your chest and upper arms, continuing to breathe deep, calming breaths centered on the diaphragm.

15. Now tense the upper back and shoulders, raising your shoulders towards your ears. Hold the tension. Now let your shoulders drop and let go of the muscles in your shoulders and upper back. You notice that your shoulders, back, abdomen, thighs, legs, and feet are heavy and relaxed.

16. Now tense the muscles of your neck and lower face, tightening your jaw, mouth, and chin. Hold it for a moment, and release the tension. Notice the difference. Let your jaw go loose so that your upper and lower teeth are not clenched. Continue to relax.

9. Now tense your forehead and eye muscles and hold the tension. Continue to breathe slowly. Now let go of the tension relaxing your forehead, eyebrows, eyes, and head. Study the feeling of relaxation in your body. As you continue to breathe slowly, you feel completely at peace and rest. Your body is heavy, almost as if it is sinking into the chair. You think about lifting your arm but it is too heavy. You are relaxed and calm.

11. As you continue to breathe, slowly begin to notice the sounds around you in the room as you remain relaxed. As I count backward in a moment you will open your eyes and return to the room feeling a continued sense of calm throughout your whole body.

    4   3   2   1   Open your eyes and stretch.

Thought Charting

Situation	Feelings	Thoughts	Re-Frame

Notes:

Session 5

Subject: Family and Others' Reaction To Your Diagnosis

Agenda:

- Have each woman select feeling words from prepared slips of paper that describe emotions of family or other relationships regarding her illness. Blank slips can be taken and filled in if there is another emotion someone wants to describe.
- Talk about the reaction of member's faith communities and select
- emotions that describe how feelings are expressed concerning their illness.
- Have discussion about the reactions of others and how it impacts the participant.
- Check on thought charting and reframing efforts.
- Practice relaxation again by initiating a brief relaxed state, then introduce guided imagery

---

Materials Needed:
1.   Slips of paper with labeled emotions (enough for each member to have a choice of at least 7) including but not limited to: *depression, guilt, anger, shock, fear, shame, helplessness.*
2.   Blank copies of thought charts with re-framing column
3.   Guided imagery script
4.   Tape of nature/ocean sounds

- Other's Reaction to Your Diagnosis

Facilitator introduces topic and passes around a basket containing feeling words on slips of paper.

Time allotted: 10 minutes

Today we're going to change our focus a little and consider the people close to you and how they have been affected by your diagnosis. Think about how the people in your life have reacted to you and to the news of your cancer. I am going to pass around a basket with slips of paper describing several emotions. Please choose one or two that seem to best describe how the people closest to you are feeling. If you have noticed a reaction that is not included, please take a blank slip of paper and write it down.

Facilitator opens the floor for discussion as soon as everyone has chosen one or two slips of paper. Encourage sharing of how the people close to participants are feeling. Facilitate understanding that the cancer is not the patient's private illness, that it affects the family/social support system in many ways. Be prepared for strong emotions and perhaps even anger that we are focusing on others who are not ill. Empathize and support responses while encouraging understanding of how the cancer affects those who are close to the participants.

Time allotted: 30 minutes

How are other people reacting to your illness?
(***Facilitator allows time for sharing.***)
How does that affect or change the way that you related before your diagnosis?
(***Facilitator allows time for sharing.***)

What types of things help you to cope with the less helpful elements of other people's emotions?
(***Facilitator allows time for sharing and reinforces positive coping responses.***)

- Checking on Reframing

Facilitator will review the thought charting exercises that have been introduced in previous sessions. Facilitator will enlist participation of the group in sharing examples of reframing and will address any difficulties that group members may be experiencing with this coping skill.

Time allotted: 20 minutes

I'd like to talk about the technique we went over last week on reframing. Please get your charts out and let's see what everyone has come up with. (***Facilitator asks for examples, stuck spots; gives feedback and guidance on reframing efforts.***)

What have you noticed about your level of emotional distress when you have successfully reframed a way of thinking about a situation?

If you are having no change in emotionality it may be that you are re-framing in a style that doesn't work for you or that there are thoughts underneath the emotion that have still not been identified. If we reframe a thought that really isn't at the core of our emotional reaction then there won't be as much difference in the way we feel. (*Facilitator asks if there are problems, examples of problems, and helps to tailor the reframing and have the member work on more thorough identification of underlying thoughts.*) Please keep tracking your emotions and thoughts so that you can get the hang of reframing. After awhile, you should be able to do this in your head and won't need to write it all out. Does anyone need new charting sheets?

- Coping Strategy: Relaxation with Guided Imagery

Facilitator introduces guided imagery as a new coping strategy and explains that this technique is added as a deeper method of relaxation. Facilitator should process the feelings of group members about this exercise before beginning and ask if anyone has tried imagery before. Fears and apprehension as well as expectations for the experience need to be addressed.

Time allotted: 20 minutes

One of the ways to ease stress in difficult life circumstances is through relaxation techniques such as the ones we have been practicing, including deep breathing and muscle relaxation. Another form of deep relaxation is called guided imagery. Guided imagery draws on your imagination to help you achieve a greater sense of calm and peace. This will involve reaching a relaxed state and imagining a peaceful place while I read a narrative helping you to imagine this kind of place. This can be a real place that you have visited or a place that you would imagine going to find quiet reflection. (*Facilitator asks if anyone in the group has tried imagery before. Negative feelings or apprehension about imagery should be discussed. **Any group member who has had a negative imagery experience, who reports a history of traumatic experiences, or who you suspect has psychopathology that will contribute to a negative experience should be allowed to remain relaxed but does not have to participate in the imagery.*)
Go ahead and get comfortable in your chairs so that we can begin the deep breathing and relaxation. Close your eyes, and focus on taking deep, relaxing breaths as we have practiced. Breath in through your nose, letting your abdomen expand, hold it for a moment, and breath out through your mouth. Continue the deep breathing as I begin to guide you into a more relaxed state. (*Facilitator uses the script for guided imagery corresponding to session 5. If possible, the lights should be dimmed during this exercise.*)

Facilitator checks in with the group to process how the imagery experience was for each person. Sharing of the experience is encouraged.

Time allotted: 10 minutes

> How are you all feeling about that exercise? Would anyone like to share how that was for you? (*Facilitator allows time for sharing and addresses any concerns such as not experiencing anything or not being able to imagine anything, Facilitator reinforces that the goal of this exercise is deep relaxation and that it is beneficial to the body. Facilitator also acknowledges that differences in experience are normal and expected.*)

Guided Imagery Exercise

(About 20 minutes)

The purpose of mental or guided imagery is to calm your body, thoughts, and emotions and to give you a break from tension and stress. This technique uses relaxation and cognition to create a relaxing place that is imagined or that you might have been and can recreate in memory.

Spend some time getting comfortable and begin your deep breathing exercises. Close your eyes and scan your body for tension. If you find tension, release it by focusing on that area and thinking the word "relax" or "calm".

As I read through a brief body scan, imagine that you are descending with each step, as if gliding down an escalator from the inside of this room to a beautiful place.

> Relax your head, forehead, face, and jaw.
> Relax your neck and shoulders.
> Relax your arms and hands.
> Relax your chest, lungs, and stomach.
> Relax your back.
> Relax your hips, legs, and feet.

Experience the relaxation and comfort present in your body as you prepare to walk out into a beautiful place. Continue to breathe slowly, in through your nose and out through your mouth and allow your breathing to become calming and rhythmic.

Though your eyes are closed, you begin to visualize the most relaxing, peaceful place that you can imagine. As the setting comes into your mind, take time to carefully notice all of the sights, sounds, smells, and sensations as if you are looking all the way around from the place in which you are standing.

Notice the colors, whether rich or muted, the vegetation, hue of any water you might see, the temperature of the air, the sounds of the environment, any textures that are near you, and any pleasant scents. As you take in the scenery, become aware of yourself in the moment. Visualize yourself with a peaceful, serene expression and take a deep breath in. As you exhale, it takes with it any tension that is left in your body. You feel completely relaxed and at peace.

In this beautiful place where you feel completely at ease and relaxed, imagine a quiet place where you can sit and enjoy your surroundings. Visualize yourself slowly walking to the place you have picked out, and sitting for awhile.

Continue to imagine yourself with a serene and pleasant expression and capture the feeling that you are in an oasis from stress and tension. Nothing can disturb you here and you are completely relaxed.

Take a few moments to enjoy the peace that exists where you are. Continue to take deep, relaxing breaths and to take in the sensory richness, letting your thoughts float by as if on a breeze, and noticing how calm you feel.

Imagine yourself rising to walk through the scene, back towards the place where you began, you are smiling, and enjoying the moment. You have found a place where you can return to anytime, and the thought is comforting.

There is a stairway close by that leads to the room where you started. You walk towards the stairs. As you climb the stairs, you will become more aware of your surroundings but will continue to feel relaxed and refreshed. You are at the bottom of the stairs now and are moving upwards. As you reach the fourth and fifth step you begin to hear the sounds in the room and become aware of what is around you. As you reach the top of the stairs you are ready to open your eyes and stretch.

Facilitator: Please process how this was for group members after the imagery. What did people enjoy about it? What types of scenes did this exercise evoke? Was it difficult for anyone to do the exercise? As with any other new skill, it can take a few practices to really relax in the exercise, and it may not be for everyone, so breathing practice with muscle relaxation can always be done for members who report not being able to imagine anything, or for whom imagery may have been negative.

Thought Charting

Situation	Feelings	Thoughts	Re-Frame

Notes:

Session 6

Subject: Self-image and Relationship with Spouse/Significant Others

Agenda

- Discussion of the effect of the diagnosis on feelings of attractiveness and how self or body image may have changed.
- Discuss the reactions of others and what are perceived as changes in the way that others relate to members as a male or female. This includes discussion of sexuality.
- Review any distressing thoughts around self-image, beliefs about attractiveness, and perception of how others see group members and practice re-framing technique.

Materials Needed:
1. Dry-erase board or flip chart and markers.
2. Guided imagery script
3. Tape of nature/ocean sounds

- Self-Image and Relationships with Others

Facilitator opens discussion by reviewing what group members were asked to reflect on during the week. Discussion about self and body image follows.

Time allotted: 15 minutes

Last week I asked you to think about how you feel about yourselves as a woman and what differences might exist in your self-image before and after your diagnosis. First, does anyone feel differently about yourself now in terms of attractiveness and self-image than you did before you learned of the cancer? ***(Facilitator allows time for sharing and validates feelings.)***

- Current or Anticipated Intimacy with a Romantic Partner

Facilitator introduces discussion topic concerning current or anticipated intimate relationships and how intimacy might be influenced by changes in the participant's body or feelings of attractiveness as a result of surgery or treatment.

Time allotted: 30 minutes

Now that you've expressed some of the feelings that you have about yourselves and some of the changes that you've experienced, consider the relationships that you have with your spouse or significant partner. How is your partner reacting to you in areas of intimacy? If you are single, how are you feeling about the possibility of a relationship?
(Facilitator allows time for discussion. Some areas may be difficult to talk about. Changes that have not yet happened may be anticipated with fear regarding attractiveness: hair loss, scar from surgery, etc.)

When you think about your spouse, partner, or the person you would want to share your life with, what qualities come to mind?
(Facilitator highlights that many of the qualities mentioned and that attract people to each other are not based on appearance.)

- Reframing: Check on Charting Self-Messages

Facilitator reinforces coping skill of thought charting by reviewing any negative self-image statements that might have been identified on thought chart. If no one has charted, facilitator can use examples discussed to write out examples of how these would be charted and reframed. Facilitator also builds empathy for how the cancer affects others by having group members brainstorm about what types of distressing thoughts or beliefs might drive reactions of significant others.

Time allotted: 15 minutes

Did anyone include feelings and beliefs about their attractiveness or self-image on the thought chart last week? *(Facilitator asks for sharing of charting examples. If none were charted, list some of the fears or apprehensions stated around self-image and turn them into core beliefs and positive reframing. Enlist help/suggestions from the group.)*

We can also use this technique to try and understand why those close to us might be reacting in certain ways. Although we don't want to try and mind-read why others act the way that they do, it might be helpful to think of other's thought processes as working in the same ways that we have talked about here. For example, if a close friend seems to avoid or change the subject when you bring up your cancer, consider the following possibilities:

Situation	Feelings	Belief
Avoiding talking about the cancer	Uncomfortable	I will say the wrong thing
	Fear	I might lose my friend

Now that you are able to make the connection between thoughts, feelings, and behavior you can understand how the people around you might be interpreting your illness. Again, we don't want to commit the "mind reading" error, just to raise the possibility that erratic or seemingly unsympathetic or even angry behavior from others can be due to underlying feelings of fear, confusion, or helplessness. In these cases, it is probably best to try some reflecting of what you think is going on so that the person in your life realizes that it is O.K. to express those deeper feelings to you.

Keeping the doors open to intimacy in communications with those close to you will help you to build and keep a vital social support system. People who have strong support systems are healthier, recover faster, and have lower rates of relapse. Even though this is an extremely trying time for you and you feel that you are the only one experiencing this, it is also a trying time for family and friends who are worried and may not want to "burden you" with their fears. Let others know that they don't have to put up a front for you and that it is normal to feel frightened, angry, and helpless.

Caregivers can be overlooked in a family member's illness and frequently suffer from anxiety and anticipatory grief. If you see signs that someone close to you is not coping with your illness very well it will be important to address so that your support system does not break down. It is not up to you to take care of everyone else at this time, but if you are sensitive to what might be going on with others around you then you might be able to steer someone towards appropriate help if needed.

- Guided Imagery

Facilitator introduces guided imagery exercise and leads group in exercise.

Time allotted: 20 minutes

I'd like to close with another exercise in guided imagery. Please get comfortable in your seats, close your eyes, and begin deep breathing. (*Facilitator reads the imagery script corresponding with session 7.*)

- Closing

Facilitator continues to prepare group for termination by alerting members that the final session is in 2 weeks. The group might want to express feelings about the ending of this process now. If not, let them know that time will be devoted next session for dealing with these issues.

Time allotted: 10 minutes

We are getting close to our last meeting so we'll be summing up what we've covered and talking about how the group experience has been for you. Think about what you feel you have gained from this experience as well as what you might not have liked about the process. Think about how you feel concerning this experience coming to a close. We will have time to talk about what this process has meant to you and about bringing things to a close.

Guided Imagery Exercise

(About 20 minutes)

The purpose of mental or guided imagery is to calm your body, thoughts, and emotions and to give you a break from tension and stress. This technique uses relaxation and cognition to create a relaxing place that is imagined or that you might have been and can recreate in memory.

Spend some time getting comfortable and begin your deep breathing exercises. Close your eyes and scan your body for tension. If you find tension, release it by focusing on that area and thinking the word "relax" or "calm".
As I read through a brief body scan, imagine that you are descending with each step, as if gliding down an escalator from the inside of this room to a beautiful place.

> Relax your head, forehead, face, and jaw.
> Relax your neck and shoulders.
> Relax your arms and hands.
> Relax your chest, lungs, and stomach.
> Relax your back.
> Relax your hips, legs, and feet.

Experience the relaxation and comfort present in your body as you prepare to walk out into a beautiful place. Continue to breathe slowly, in through your nose and out through your mouth and allow your breathing to become calming and rhythmic.

Though your eyes are closed, you begin to visualize the most relaxing, peaceful place that you can imagine. As the setting comes into your mind, take time to carefully notice all of the sights, sounds, smells, and sensations as if you are looking all the way around from the place in which you are standing.

Notice the colors, whether rich or muted, the vegetation, hue of any water you might see, the temperature of the air, the sounds of the environment, any textures that are near you, and any pleasant scents. As you take in the scenery, become aware of yourself in the moment. Visualize yourself with a peaceful, serene expression and take a deep breath in. As you exhale, it takes with it any tension that is left in your body. You feel completely relaxed and at peace.

In this beautiful place where you feel completely at ease and relaxed, imagine a quiet place where you can sit and enjoy your surroundings. Visualize yourself slowly walking to the place you have picked out, and sitting for awhile.

Continue to imagine yourself with a serene and pleasant expression and capture the feeling that you are in an oasis from stress and tension. Nothing can disturb you here and you are completely relaxed.

Take a few moments to enjoy the peace that exists where you are. Continue to take deep, relaxing breaths and to take in the sensory richness, letting your thoughts float by as if on a breeze, and noticing how calm you feel.

Imagine yourself rising to walk through the scene, back towards the place where you began, you are smiling, and enjoying the moment. You have found a place where you can return to anytime, and the thought is comforting.

There is a stairway close by that leads to the room where you started. You walk towards the stairs. As you climb the stairs, you will become more aware of your surroundings but will continue to feel relaxed and refreshed. You are at the bottom of the stairs now and are moving upwards. As you reach the fourth and fifth step you begin to hear the sounds in the room and become aware of what is around you. As you reach the top of the stairs you are ready to open your eyes and stretch.

Facilitator: Please process how this was for group members after the imagery. What did people enjoy about it? What types of scenes did this exercise evoke? Was it difficult for anyone to do the exercise? As with any other new skill, it can take a few practices to really relax in the exercise, and it may not be for everyone, so breathing practice with muscle relaxation can always be done for members who report not being able to imagine anything, or for whom imagery may have been negative.

Session 7

Subject: Establish New Goals

Agenda:

- Identifying reasons for living and conceptualizing these as life goals.
- Set short (6-month) and long-term (1 to 3 year) goals and address feelings related to cancer and ability to reach goals.
- Examine existential goals or those in spiritual/faith life and whether goals/priorities have changed as a result of the diagnosis.
- Repeat guided imagery exercise

Materials Needed
1. Dry-erase board or flip chart and markers.
2. Worksheets for short- and long-term goals.

- Setting Life Goals: Reasons For Living

Facilitator introduces topic of goal setting by talking about how having reasons for living can help in coping with illness.

Time allotted: 10 minutes

As we've talked during the last few sessions you've been able to learn about and discuss different ways to cope with your illness. You've been able to see how taking an active role in the way you think about and react to situations can ease some of the difficulty. You've practiced relaxation and imagery and have identified feelings that you and others have about your diagnosis. All of these strategies are important for helping you to feel a sense of control and coping during this time in your life.

Today, we're going to move from a sense of control to a sense of <u>purpose</u>. What I'd like for you to do today is think about what gets you up in the morning; the reasons you have for living. These can be very personal such as children, family, pets, or things you want to see happen in your life; they can have professional aspects such as career or academic goals; they can even be tangible such as a home. Take a few minutes to think about the reasons for living that are important to you.

(Facilitator allows about 3 minutes for members to think about reasons.)

Who would like to begin sharing some of the reasons for living that are important to you?
(Facilitator listens and allows time for sharing. As group shares reasons, facilitator writes them on the board or easel. The purpose of this is to identify common threads among group members such as family or other reasons.)

Facilitator now leads the group to frame purposes as life goals. Address any resistance to setting long-term goals. It is common for many cancer patients to have fears of not being alive to reach long-term goals. If no one voices this fear but some in the group are silent, be prepared to address the fear of dying out loud to open conversation. This can be compassionately introduced in a reflection stating that sometimes people with cancer are afraid to make long term plans because they don't' know whether they will "make it" and by asking if this is what anyone in the group is thinking.

Time allotted: 50 minutes

Let's look at the reasons in the form of goals. Some will be short-term goals and others will be more long-term goals. Look at this list of reasons and think about how to make them into goal statements. What might you be feeling or thinking about setting life goals?
(Facilitator allows a few moments and addresses silence or expressed fears by talking about the fear of dying. Facilitator should normalize this fear as an expected reaction considering the diagnosis and experience of cancer.)
The reason we are including goal setting as a part of coping strategies is that goals and plans give you a reason to live and a reason to take care of yourself by adhering to treatment and self-care. Goals also give you something to look forward to. Goals help to redirect energy that might otherwise be expended on worry about prognosis or recovery so much that you feel hopeless and abandon previous interests and plans. Renewing previous interests, setting goals, making plans, and having something to look forward to can be a coping strength.

What would you like to accomplish in the next six months?
Discuss.

What kinds of goals can you set for the next year and for the future?
Discuss.

What I'd like you to do now is to make a contract with yourselves that will affirm your reasons for living and help you to focus your energy on achieving your goals. I am going to pass around goal worksheet forms for you to fill out. These are for you to keep and refer to whenever you need them.
(Facilitator passes around worksheets and instructs members to think about and filling in the columns for short and long-term goals during the next week.)

- Guided Imagery: Achieving Goals

Facilitator introduces guided imagery

Time allotted: 20 minutes

Now that you have spelled out your goals, it is important for you to be able to visualize yourselves reaching them. We are going to return to the guided imagery exercise from last week. Go ahead and begin by getting comfortable in your seats, close your eyes, and start breathing deep, relaxing breaths.
(Facilitator will talk the group through a few minutes of deep breathing and will then follow the guided imagery script for session 6.)

Facilitator continues to prepare group members for termination of the group by addressing that there is only one sessions remaining. Facilitator also reminds group to review thought charting and gives next week's topic for reflection.

Time allotted: 5 minutes

Next week will be our last session. You will all have time to share what you have gained from the group, and what you might take with you as a result of participation. It is also important to discuss expectations that might not have been met through the group or things you would have liked to have spent more or less time on.   It is important to recognize our time together, and to talk about what it means for everyone to end our time as a group.

- Closing

Guided Imagery Exercise

(About 20 minutes)

The purpose of mental or guided imagery is to calm your body, thoughts, and emotions and to give you a break from tension and stress. This technique uses relaxation and cognition to create a relaxing place that is imagined or that you might have been and can recreate in memory.

Spend some time getting comfortable and begin your deep breathing exercises. Close your eyes and scan your body for tension. If you find tension, release it by focusing on that area and thinking the word "relax" or "calm".
As I read through a brief body scan, imagine that you are descending with each step, as if gliding down an escalator from the inside of this room to a beautiful place.

> Relax your head, forehead, face, and jaw.
> Relax your neck and shoulders.
> Relax your arms and hands.
> Relax your chest, lungs, and stomach.
> Relax your back.
> Relax your hips, legs, and feet.

Experience the relaxation and comfort present in your body as you prepare to walk out into a beautiful place. Continue to breathe slowly, in through your nose and out through your mouth and allow your breathing to become calming and rhythmic.

Though your eyes are closed, you begin to visualize the most relaxing, peaceful place that you can imagine. As the setting comes into your mind, take time to carefully notice all of the sights, sounds, smells, and sensations as if you are looking all the way around from the place in which you are standing.

Notice the colors, whether rich or muted, the vegetation, hue of any water you might see, the temperature of the air, the sounds of the environment, any textures that are near you, and any pleasant scents. As you take in the scenery, become aware of yourself in the moment. Visualize yourself with a peaceful, serene expression and take a deep breath in. As you exhale, it takes with it any tension that is left in your body. You feel completely relaxed and at peace.

In this beautiful place where you feel completely at ease and relaxed, imagine a quiet place where you can sit and enjoy your surroundings. Visualize yourself slowly walking to the place you have picked out, and sitting for awhile.

Continue to imagine yourself with a serene and pleasant expression and capture the feeling that you are in an oasis from stress and tension. Nothing can disturb you here and you are completely relaxed.

Take a few moments to enjoy the peace that exists where you are. Continue to take deep, relaxing breaths and to take in the sensory richness, letting your thoughts float by as if on a breeze, and noticing how calm you feel.

Imagine yourself rising to walk through the scene, back towards the place where you began, you are smiling, and enjoying the moment. You have found a place where you can return to anytime, and the thought is comforting.

There is a stairway close by that leads to the room where you started. You walk towards the stairs. As you climb the stairs, you will become more aware of your surroundings but will continue to feel relaxed and refreshed. You are at the bottom of the stairs now and are moving upwards. As you reach the fourth and fifth step you begin to hear the sounds in the room and become aware of what is around you. As you reach the top of the stairs you are ready to open your eyes and stretch.

Facilitator: Please process how this was for group members after the imagery. What did people enjoy about it? What types of scenes did this exercise evoke? Was it difficult for anyone to do the exercise? As with any other new skill, it can take a few practices to really relax in the exercise, and it may not be for everyone, so breathing practice with muscle relaxation can always be done for members who report not being able to imagine anything, or for whom imagery may have been negative.

Goals: Reasons for Living

These are the goals I am setting for the future. They are about relationships, activities, hobbies, interests, plans, or things that are important to me.

SHORT-TERM GOALS: IN NEXT 3-6 MONTHS

LONG-TERM GOALS

Session 8

Subject: Summing Up

Agenda:

- Review skills covered and discuss what was most helpful and least helpful for each member
- Process feelings about the group ending
- Discuss social and religious supports and how members plan to maintain coping skills.
- Assess the need for referrals for continued psychological services

Materials Needed:
1. Referral numbers for those requiring additional therapy.
2. Patient Satisfaction Survey

- Summing Up

Facilitator reviews the skills covered in the last 7 sessions and invites the group to share what they have found most/least helpful throughout the process. This helps to consolidate the gains that members have made in building their coping skills. Discussion should also focus on saying goodbye by talking about what members will miss from sharing this time together. This will help members to process feelings about the group ending.

Time allotted: 60 minutes

In the last seven meetings we have covered several techniques of coping that were included to help give you the best possible tools for dealing with your diagnosis. We have practiced breathing, muscle relaxation, and guided imagery. You have learned how your thoughts, beliefs, and feelings are connected and how to catch yourself when you are thinking in ways that are not helpful to you. You've been able to identify and share your emotions with others and have explored what people close to you might be feeling.

What do you feel has been the most helpful part of this experience?
(Discuss.)
What do you feel was least helpful?

(Discuss.)

How are you feeling about the group ending?
(Discuss.)

How do you plan to keep the positive steps you've made after you leave here today?
(Discuss and reinforce plans of social connectedness and practice of skills.)

- Closing

Facilitator thanks group for their participation and offers to provide numbers and referrals for anyone who feels that they would like additional counseling. Facilitator closes the session with prayer in an unstructured form or uses guidelines provided

Time allotted: 15 minutes

I want to thank you all for agreeing to be a part of this group and for sharing so much with me and with the other group members. Your participation has been a valuable part of the process and is greatly appreciated. It is normal to feel sad and a little apprehensive about the group ending, but if you are feeling concern over your level of distress about group ending at this point please see me after we finish and we'll talk about some options for you.

Participant Satisfaction Survey

Please rate your experience as part of the group by answering the following questions. Feel free to elaborate when appropriate in the spaces provided.

1. The convenience of the location for group sessions.
0	1	2	3	4	5
not helpful			neutral		very helpful

2. The introductory talk on coping to your decision to participate.
0	1	2	3	4	5
not helpful			neutral		very helpful

3. The explanation of the study during the initial questionnaire answer session.
0	1	2	3	4	5
not helpful			neutral		very helpful

4. Meeting with the group therapist and/or co-therapist prior to the first session.
0	1	2	3	4	5
not helpful			neutral		very helpful

5. The characteristics of the group leader.
0	1	2	3	4	5
not helpful			neutral		very helpful

   Please explain:_____
   _____
   _____

6. The presence of others who have also been diagnosed with breast cancer.
0	1	2	3	4	5
not helpful			neutral		very helpful

7. The relaxation, deep breathing, and guided imagery exercises.
0	1	2	3	4	5
not helpful			neutral		very helpful

8. The thought-charting and thinking style awareness exercises.

   0   1   2   3   4   5

   not helpful   neutral   very helpful

9. The sessions where we talked about feelings and reactions of family.

   0   1   2   3   4   5

   not helpful   neutral   very helpful

10. If applicable, the inclusion of faith as a coping resource.

    0   1   2   3   4   5

About the author

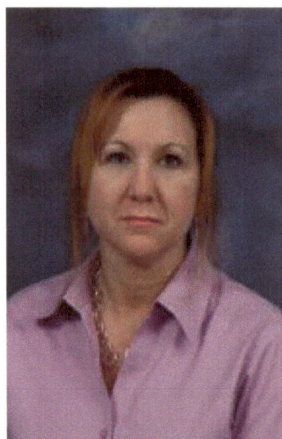

Stacey Scott is a Licensed Clinical Psychologist practicing in Virginia. She received her Doctorate in Clinical Psychology degree from Regent University in 2003 and was awarded Outstanding Graduate of her program. Dr. Scott has served as Adjunct Faculty for the Clinical Psychology Doctoral Program at Regent as well as teaching continuing education sessions locally and nationally. She designed her agency's internship training program and obtained APPIC-member status for the program in 2003. Dr. Scott served as the Clinical Training Director of the Pre-Doctoral Internship in Clinical Psychology at Eden Family Institute from 2005-2007.

Dr. Scott worked as the Director of FirstFruits Crisis Response team from December of 2001 through August of 2007 and has been trained in Critical Incident Stress Management and Debriefing as well as obtaining Red Cross Disaster Mental Health certification. She coordinated and worked on dozens of mental health relief and intervention trips to New York City following September 11th, 2001 and continues to work locally and nationally in disaster mental health services as well as intervening when other types of trauma affect communities.

Her work with cancer and serious illness began long before her career as a psychologist with training and volunteer companion work at Full Circle Aids Hospice. Dr. Scott designed and completed a pilot study of group therapy with breast cancer patients at Virginia Beach General Hospital which was the basis of her doctoral dissertation. She is currently President of the Southeastern Virginia division of the National Ovarian Cancer Coalition and is working to increase education and awareness of ovarian cancer in that region. Dr. Scott is presently working with senior adults in assisted living facilities across Southwestern Virginia providing assessments as well as psychological and behavioral health services.

Dr. Scott is married and resides in Southampton County, Virginia with her husband, Marshall Swink, their Labrador retriever Seyval, and Claude, a cantankerous Maine Coon cat.